Blood Type O – Cookbook

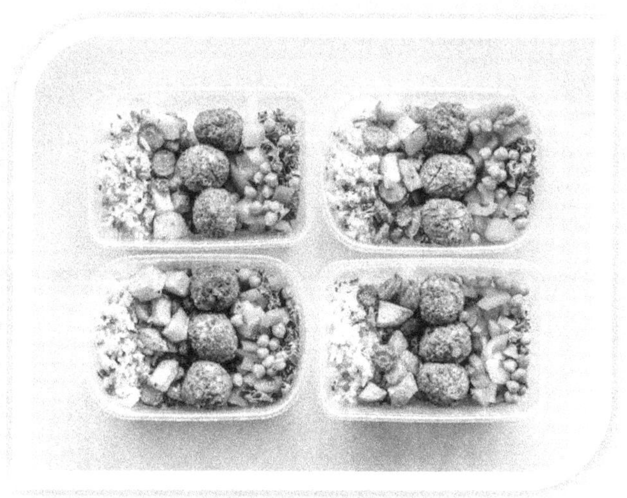

60 Easy Nutritious Recipes for Your Blood Type to Maintain Optimal Health

ALVIN LEWIS

Copyright © 2023 by ALVIN LEWIS

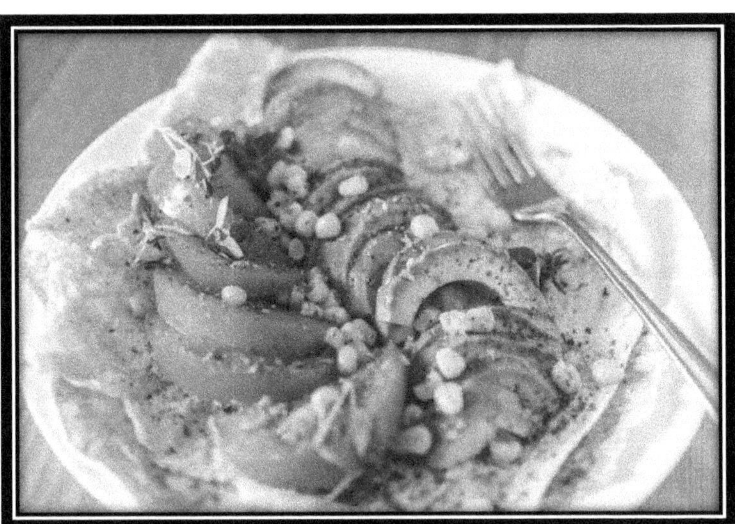

Table of contents

Other Books by the Author

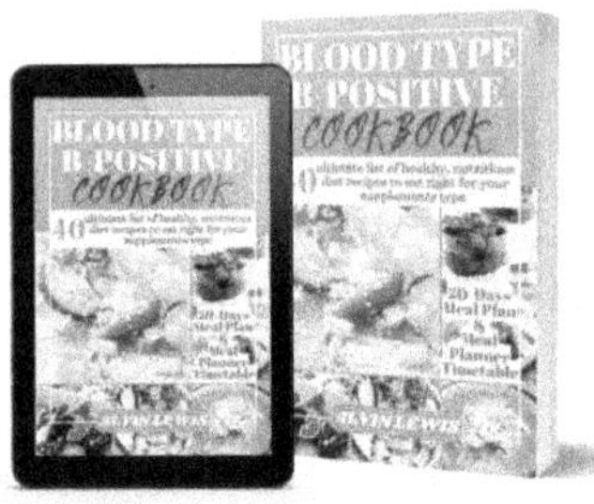

BLOOD TYPE B-POSITIVE COOKBOOK

ALSO CHECK OUT MORE BOOKS BY ALVIN LEWIS

SCAN THE QR CODE BELOW

Introduction

Welcome to The Blood Type O Cookbook, a gastronomic journey beyond the ordinary. We cordially encourage you to discover the secrets of a dynamic and customized lifestyle designed especially for blood type O individuals in your pursuit of optimal health. This cookbook is more than simply a list of recipes; it's your passport to a more vibrant, energized, and healthy version of yourself.

Meet Maya who lived in the center of a busy metropolis, whose journey towards a healthier lifestyle was shaped through the simple profound decisions she made every day. Maya, who has blood type O, learned the significant benefits of eating a diet customized to meet her individual requirements.

During a routine checkup, Maya discovered the blood type diet, which marked the beginning of her awakening. She was intrigued and did some research, finding that people with blood type O thrived well on a diet high in protein. The revelation prompted her to change her eating habits, embracing lean meats, fish, and veggies in place of processed meals.

As Maya started her nutritional journey, the improvements were evident. Her complexion shone, she had more energy, and her digestion even became better. Maya's body yearned for the vital nutrition it needed, so each morning she began with a substantial breakfast of eggs and spinach. Dinner and lunch were a colorful array of vibrant vegetables and lean meats, a symphony of flavors that nourished her from the inside out.

Her friends noticed the transformation and were excited to accompany her on her journey to wellness. Maya turned into an inspiration to everyone around her, imparting her wisdom and experiences. They came together as a community and supported one another to make healthier choices.

Maya's story was a testament to the power of understanding one's unique needs and making informed choices. With each passing day, she radiated vitality, proving that a harmonious balance of nutrition and community could truly unlock the doors to a healthier and happier life.

Understanding your individual biological composition is the first step to maximizing your health. Blood type O individuals are known for specific traits that influence how their bodies respond to food. People with blood type O, who have been historically associated with hunter-gatherer origins, are thought to do well on a diet high in fruits, vegetables, and lean proteins. This cookbook unlocks a world of benefits from improved energy levels to a faster metabolism by catering to these particular dietary requirements.

As you delve into the pages of the Blood Type O Cookbook, anticipate discovering a variety of mouthwatering recipes meticulously curated to suit your blood type. Every meal, from filling dinners to substantial breakfast choices, is not only a pleasure to the taste sensations but also a step toward realizing the potential of your body.

Come embrace a way of living that goes beyond traditional diets, where each meal is an intentional decision to nourish your body according to your blood type. Prepare to experience the flavors of vitality and set out on a life-changing path that will lead to a healthier, more energetic version of yourself. The Blood Type O Cookbook is your partner in the quest for optimal health, not just a reference.

How Diet Can Impact Blood Type

Understanding the relationship between our diet and health and how it interacts with our blood type reveals a significant aspect of customized nutrition. According to recent research, people with different blood types may react differently to different foods, which can have an impact on our energy levels, metabolism, and general vitality in addition to our physical health.

Blood Type O individuals, who are frequently identified as the ancestors' hunter-gatherer blood type, are most affected by nutrition. It is thought that our genetic makeup and nutritional requirements are related. Therefore, the Blood Type O diet emphasizes lean proteins, lots of vegetables, and some fruits, which is consistent with the diets that early hunter-gatherer societies are said to have followed.

Investigating the complex relationship between blood type and nutrition provides access to customized nutrition. It enables people to make deliberate decisions that are in line with their own physiological make-up. Blood type and food interact to potentially unlock personalized wellbeing, from affecting digestion to maybe reducing the chance of certain health issues.

The Blood Type O Cookbook proves to be an invaluable resource as we set out on this understanding journey, including meals that have been carefully selected to meet the dietary requirements of those who identify as Blood Type O.

This investigation goes beyond general dietary recommendations, ushering in a time where every meal is a conscious choice towards overall wellbeing. It's intriguing to consider how diet affects blood type since it can help us reevaluate how we eat and start living a more vibrant, healthy life.

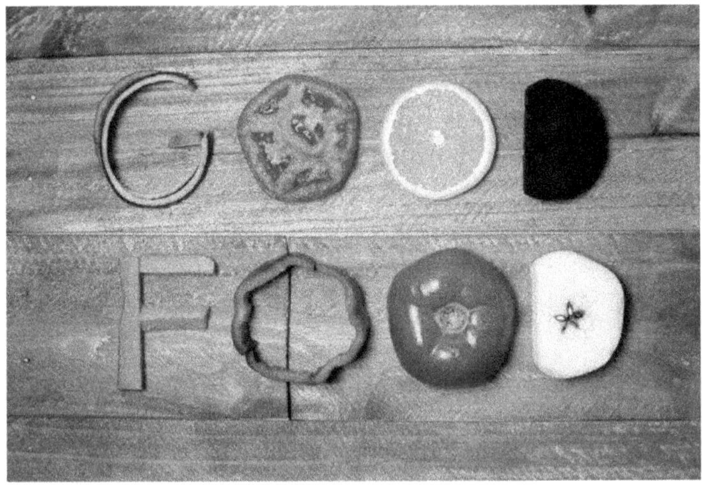

Chapter 1: Understanding Blood Type O Diet

Overview of Blood Type O Characteristics

Blood type O is a distinct chapter in the intricate tapestry of human biology, impacting not only our circulatory system but also providing information on a range of physiological traits. Knowing the unique characteristics of Blood Type O paints a picture of tenacity, flexibility, and ancestry that influences dietary and lifestyle suggestions.

1. The Tradition of Hunter-Gatherer: Because blood type O is thought to have genetic ties to early hunter-gatherer populations, it is sometimes referred to as the "hunter-gatherer" blood type. It is thought that this ancestry influences a number of nutrition and health-related factors.

2. Strong Digestive System: Blood type O individuals are believed to have a strong and effective digestive system. This trait is consistent with the historical function of hunter-gatherers, who relied on a wide variety of foods to survive.

3. The Aspect of Metabolism: One of the main characteristics of Blood Type O is said to be metabolism, which is essential to general health. Blood type-based diet proponents contend that eating a diet specific to one's blood type can enhance metabolic functions and may have an effect on weight management.

4. Stress Resilience: Blood Type O individuals are frequently linked to stress resilience. This resilience is thought to have its roots in the difficulties that our early hunter-gatherer ancestors experienced, which called for flexibility and quick thinking in a variety of settings.

Knowing these traits lays the foundations for customizing lifestyle decisions, especially when it comes to food and fitness. With recipes designed to complement these innate characteristics, The Blood Type O Cookbook acts as a helpful manual, enabling people to make decisions that are in line with their own biology. We set out on a voyage of self-discovery as we explore the traits of Blood Type O and realize the depth that individualized wellness may offer to our existence.

Dietary Recommendations for Blood Type O

Given that blood type O is frequently linked to "hunter-gatherer" origins, people with this blood type may do well on a diet similar to that of early humans. Although specific requirements may differ, the following basic dietary guidelines are specific to blood type O.

1. Proteins Consumption: People with blood type O are frequently advised to prioritize animal proteins since they are thought to be more closely associated with the diet of ancestors. Lean meats such as fish, chicken, and lean red meat can be included in regular meals. To guarantee a well-balanced diet, it is imperative to select high-quality, organic sources whenever feasible.

2. Vegetables: Emphasize the need of eating a range of vegetables, especially cruciferous and leafy greens. These supply vital nutrients, vitamins, and fiber. Including a diverse range of vibrant vegetables helps improve general health and wellbeing.

Grains and Legumes: Individuals with blood type O may benefit from consuming fewer grains and legumes because these foods contain lectins, which may not be compatible to their digestive tracts. Instead, choose grains free of gluten, such as quinoa and rice, in moderation.

Fruits: Focus on fruits that are low in lectins, which can impede digestion, and high in antioxidants. In general, berries, cherries, and plums are well-tolerated. Individuals should, however, be aware of how they personally react to different fruits and modify their consumption accordingly.

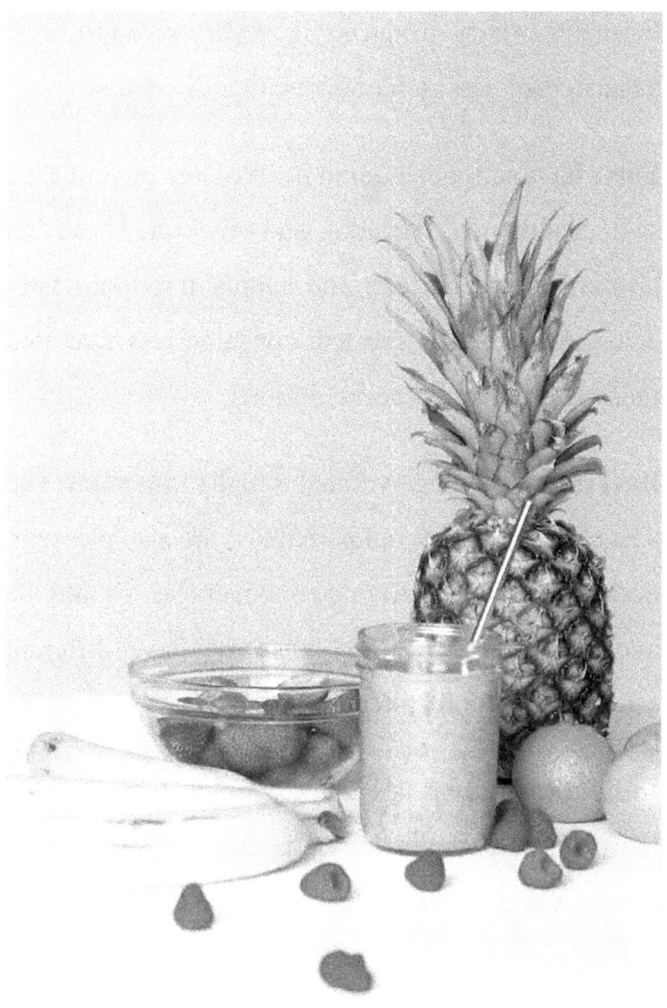

Dairy: It is advisable to choose dairy products that are easily digestible and low in fat, even though they are not completely forbidden.

Fermented dairy products, like kefir or yogurt, may be easier for certain blood type O individuals.

Fats: Include foods high in healthy fats in your diet, such as almonds, avocados, and olive oil. These fats promote general health and supply important fatty acids. Avoids trans fats and consume less saturated fat from fried and processed foods.

Beverages: Staying hydrated is really important. The best choice is water, but herbal teas are also pleasant. Sodas and other caffeinated beverages should be avoided or limited since they may have different effects on those with blood type O.

Individual Variations: It's crucial to note that individual responses to foods can vary. Although these suggestions offer a broad framework, individuals should pay attention to their own bodies and modify according to their particular requirements and preferences.

Benefits of Following Blood Type O Diet

For those with blood type O, there are many advantages to following a diet specific to their blood type. It can be a life-changing experience. Although individual reactions to dietary modifications may differ, the following is a thorough look of possible benefits of adhering to the Blood Type O diet.

1. Optimized Metabolism: The Blood Type O diet fits the supposed "hunter-gatherer" ancestral profile linked to this blood type. By emphasizing lean proteins and reducing certain lectin-rich food, this diet may help maintain an optimal metabolism, which can help with weight control and overall energy levels.

2. Improved Digestive Wellbeing: Dietary planning for blood type O involves a focus on meals that are good for the digestive system. This can lead to improved gut health, reduced bloating, and better nutrient absorption, promoting a healthier digestive environment.

3. Enhanced Energy Levels: For those with blood type O, a diet high in lean proteins and nutrient-dense vegetables may provide them with continuous energy throughout the day. Following this diet can help people feel more energized and alert because it eliminates foods that may trigger energy slumps.

4. Enhanced Immune Response: Consuming food thought to support the immune system is encouraged by the Blood Type O diet. Premium proteins when paired with nutrient-dense fruits and vegetables provide vital vitamins and minerals that can strengthen and support the immune system.

5. Balanced Blood Sugar: A focus on lean proteins and a decrease in foods high in lectins could help improve blood sugar regulation. Individuals with blood type O may benefit the most from this, since it may lower their chance of developing insulin resistance and improve their general metabolic health.

6. Improved Mental Sharpness: A diet high in vital nutrients and well-balanced can benefit cognitive performance. Some Blood Type O diet adherents claim increased mental acuity, concentration, and general wellbeing.

7. Decreased Inflammation: People with blood type O may have lower levels of inflammation in their bodies by avoiding foods that can cause inflammation. Given the numerous health problems linked to persistent inflammation, this could have far-reaching effects.

8. Customized Nutritional Approach: The customized nature of the Blood Type O diet is one of its distinctive features. This diet offers a framework for customizing nutrition to meet individual needs, acknowledging that people may react differently to different foods. This approach promotes self-determination and control over one's health.

It's critical to keep an open mind when implementing the Blood Type O diet and to acknowledge that every person will react differently. While some people might gain a lot, others might not have the same results. As with any dietary adjustment, seeking the advice of a nutritionist or healthcare provider can yield tailored recommendations based on a person's unique needs and objectives.

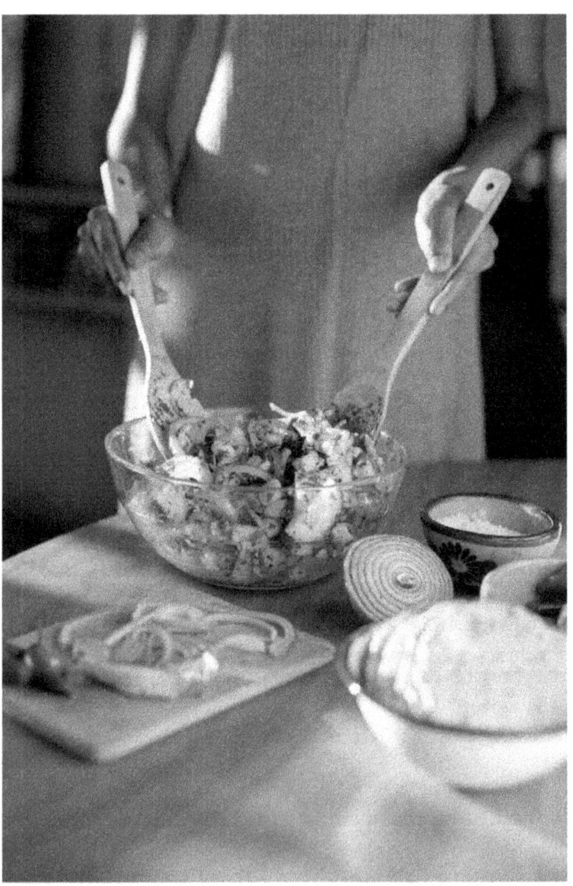

Chapter 2: Stocking Your Blood Type O Kitchen

Essential Ingredients for Blood Type O Diet

When following the Blood Type O diet to achieve optimal health, choosing the right ingredients is essential to creating meals that suit the specific traits of this blood type. These fundamental components, which range from nutrient-rich veggies to lean proteins, serve as the foundation for a meal that is intended to improve health and vigor.

1. Lean Protein: Rich, lean proteins are the foundation of the Blood Type O diet. Embrace sources such as poultry, turkey, lamb, and lean beef. These proteins promote muscle growth and metabolic efficiency in addition to fitting with the diet that early hunter-gatherers are thought to have consumed.

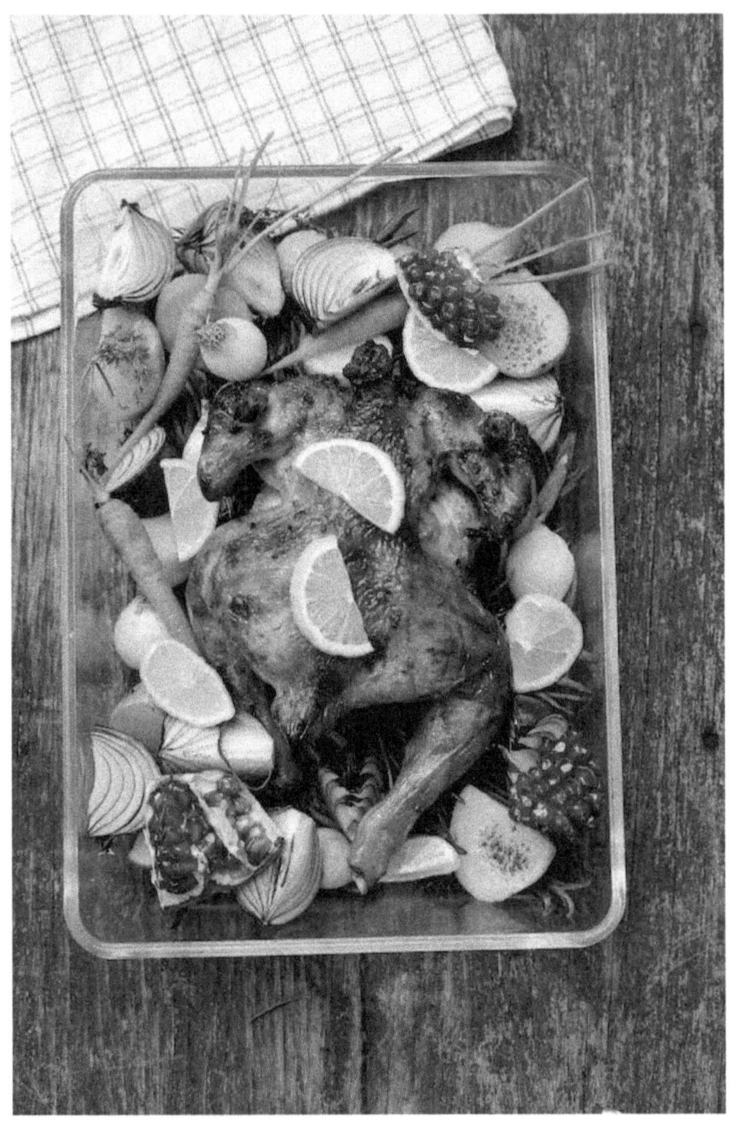

2. An abundance of veggies: A Blood Type O diet is centered on dark, leafy greens. Broccoli, kale, and spinach are full of phytonutrients and antioxidants that support healthy digestion and general health. Incorporate a vibrant assortment of veggies to optimize the nutritious content.

3. Conceivable Fruits: Certain fruits should be consumed in moderation, but others should only be eaten infrequently. Figs, plums, and berries are considered beneficial for those with Blood Type O. These fruits offer vital vitamins and antioxidants in addition to a hint of sweetness.

4. Limited Grains and Quinoa: Whole grain like quinoa are great sources of complex carbohydrates for sustained energy. Nonetheless, the Blood Type O diet suggests limiting the intake of specific grains, highlighting the necessity for substitutes that correspond with this blood type's digestive traits.

5. Nutritious Fats: Incorporate sources of healthy fats in your food, such as almonds, flaxseed oil, and olive oil. These fats balance out the Blood Type O diet's emphasis on proteins by promoting heart health and satisfaction.

6. Fish and Seafood: Heart health and general well-being are enhanced by the important omega-3 fatty acids found in fatty fish like mackerel and salmon. Seafood and fish contribute a savory element to the diet and help meet Blood Type O's nutritional requirements.

Kitchen Tools and Equipment

Embarking on the enriching journey of the Blood Type O diet requires not only the proper ingredients but also the right tools to turn them into nourishing, tasty meals. These kitchen appliances and tools are crucial when creating a diet that complements the traits of Blood Type O Individuals, from effective meal planning to thoughtful cooking methods.

1. Superior Blender: A good blender is a useful tool for making healthy drinks and smoothies that are high in nutrients. A blender makes sure that the abundance of fruits and vegetables that are recommended in the Blood Type O diet are smooth and readily absorbed.

2. Stainless Steel Cookware: Invest in durable cookware made of stainless steel to prepare lean proteins and sauté veggies. Stainless steel is a simple material to maintain and offers a dependable and secure cooking surface that aligns with the guidelines of the Blood Type O diet.

3. Sharp Chef's Knife: Cutting through a wide range of materials, such as lean meats and vibrant vegetables, requires a sharp chef's knife. Chopping with precision maximizes nutrient retention and improves the cooking process as a whole.

4. Steamer Basket: In the Blood Type O diet, steaming is the ideal way of cooking since it maintains the nutritional value of vegetables. Vegetables with intrinsic health advantages can be prepared with ease and bright color thanks to a steamer basket.

5. High-Grade Cutting Board: A durable cutting board is a need in the kitchen when preparing meals. When cutting items, use a board made of food-safe plastic or bamboo to keep things hygienic and avoid cross-contamination.

6. Food Processor: A food processor simplifies the process of making sauces, dressings, and nut butters—elements that give Blood Type O meals taste and nutritional value. To make a variety of cooking activities easier, look for a food processor that is multifunctional.

7. BBQ Pan or Grill: For Blood Type O individuals, grilling is a favored cooking method, especially for lean meats. Invest in barbecue or a grill pan so you can cook indoors all year long and reap the benefits of this method.

Having these basic items in your kitchen not only makes cooking more enjoyable, but it also ensures that Blood Type O meal preparation follows the guidelines of tailored nutrition.

Chapter 3: Breakfast Delights

1. Hearty Omelette with Turkey and Vegetable

Ingredients:

- 3 big eggs

- 1/4 cup chopped bell peppers

- 1/4 cup diced turkey

- 1/4 cup chopped spinach

- 1 tablespoon olive oil

- Salt and pepper to taste

Guidelines:

In a bowl, whisk the eggs until well beaten thoroughly. In a non-stick pan, warm the olive oil over medium heat. Add the spinach, bell peppers, and turkey to the pan and sauté the vegetables until they are soft. Drizzle the whisked eggs over the vegetables. Cook until the omelette's edges are firm, then carefully raise it and fold it in half. Continue cooking the eggs until they are completely set. To taste, add salt and pepper for seasoning.

2. Porridge with Quinoa and Berries

Ingredients:

- 1/2 cup quinoa

- 1/2 cup mixed berries (strawberries, raspberries, and blueberries)

- 1 cup almond milk

- 1/4 teaspoon vanilla extract

- 1 tablespoon honey

- Chopped nuts (optional) as a garnish

Guidelines:

Give the quinoa a good rinse in cold water. Put the quinoa and almond milk in a saucepan. Once the quinoa reaches a boiling point, lower the heat to a simmer and let it cook for 15 minutes or until it's cooked. Add vanilla extract and honey, and stir.

To serve, ladle the porridge into dishes, sprinkle with mixed berries and garnish with chopped nuts if preferred.

3. Mushroom Frittata and Spinach

Ingredients:

- 4 big eggs

- 1/2 cup of sliced mushrooms

- 1 cup chopped spinach

- 1/4 cup of chopped onions

- 1/4 cup of Parmesan cheese, grated

- To taste, add salt and pepper.

- 1 tablespoon of olive oil.

Guidelines:

Turn the oven on to 350°F (175°C). Whisk the eggs in a bowl and add pepper and salt to taste. In an oven-safe skillet, heat the olive oil over medium heat. Sauté mushrooms and onions until softened. Add spinach then cook to wilt.

Drizzle the whisked eggs over the vegetables in the skillet. Top the eggs with a sprinkle of Parmesan cheese. Move the skillet to the preheated oven and bake the frittata for 15 to 20 minutes, or until it sets.

4. Energizing Green Smoothie

Ingredients:

- 1 cup of stem-free kale leaves

- 1/2 banana

- 1/2 cup pineapple chunks

- 1/2 cup sliced and peeled cucumber

- 1/2 cup coconut water

- Ice cubes, if desired

Guidelines:

Put kale, banana, pineapple, cucumber, and coconut water in a blender. Blend until smooth. Add ice cubes, if preferred then blend again. Transfer to a glass and savor this cool green smoothie.

5. Buckwheat Pancakes with Mixed Berries

Ingredients:

- 1 tablespoon baking powder

- 1 cup buckwheat flour

- A tsp. honey

- 1 cup almond milk

- 1 egg

- 1/2 cup mixed berries

- Coconut oil for cooking

Guidelines:

In a bowl, whisk together almond milk, egg, honey, baking powder, and buckwheat flour until smooth. In a skillet, warm the coconut oil over a medium heat. To form little pancakes, pour batter into the skillet. Cook until surface bubbles appear, then turn and cook the other side. Garnish with a mixture of berries.

6. Turkey and Avocado Wrap

Ingredients:

- 1 whole grain wrap

- 1/2 avocado, sliced

- 3 turkey slices

- Handful of spinach leaves

- 1 tablespoon Greek yogurt

- To taste, add salt and pepper

Guidelines:

Place the whole grain wrap onto a level surface. Cover the wrap with Greek yogurt. Arrange spinach leaves, avocado slices, and turkey slices in layers. Add pepper and salt for seasoning. Tightly roll the wrap, then slice in half.

7. Berry Parfait with Quinoa

Ingredients:

- 1/2 cup greek yogurt

- 1/2 cup cooked quinoa

- 1/2 cup mixed berries (blueberries, strawberries)

- 1 tablespoon honey

- Chopped nuts as garnish (optional)

Guidelines:

Layer Greek yogurt, cooked quinoa, and mixed berries in a glass. Drizzle with honey over top. Repeat the layers again. If preferred, garnish with chopped nuts.

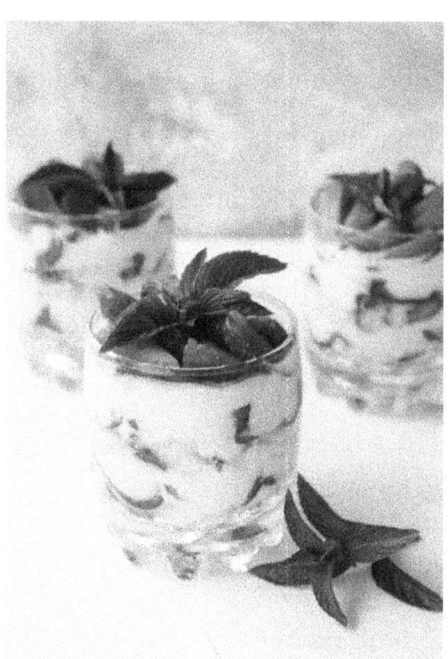

8. Chia Seed Pudding with Almond Milk

Ingredients:

- 3 tablespoons chia seeds

- 1 cup almond milk

- 1 tablespoon maple syrup

- 1/2 teaspoon vanilla extract

- Sliced banana as garnish

Guidelines:

Mix chia seeds, almond milk, maple syrup, and vanilla extract in a bowl. Give it a good stir, then refrigerate for at least 2 hours or overnight. Stir the pudding and top with sliced banana before serving.

9. Turkey and Vegetables Breakfast Burrito

Ingredients:

- 1 whole grain tortilla

- 2 scrambled eggs

- 1/4 cup chopped bell peppers

- 1/4 cup diced turkey

- Salsa as topping

- Fresh cilantro for garnish

Guidelines:

Sauté the diced turkey and bell peppers in a skillet until cooked. Add the scrambled eggs to the skillet and cook through until eggs are set. Heat the whole grain tortilla. Spoon the tortilla with the egg and turkey mixture. Add salsa to top and sprinkle fresh cilantro to garnish. Roll into a burrito and savor it.

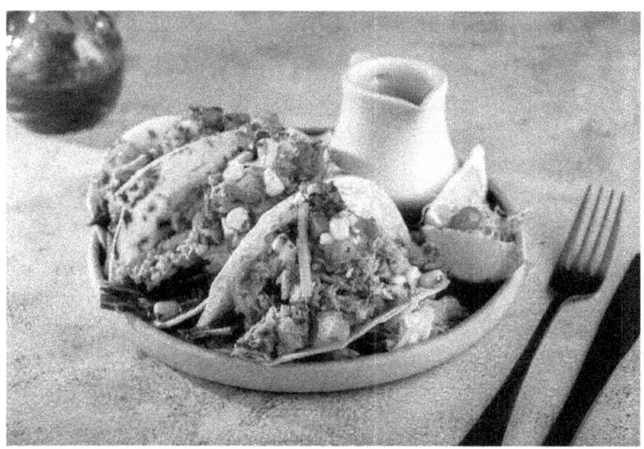

10. Blueberry Almond Smoothie Bowl

Ingredients:

- 1 cup blueberries, frozen

- 1/2 banana

- 2 tablespoons almond butter

- 1/2 cup almond milk

- Garnish with sliced almond, chia seeds and fresh blueberries.

Guidelines:

In a blender put frozen blueberries, banana, almond milk, and almond butter. Blend until smooth. Transfer the blended smoothie to a bowl. Top with fresh blueberries, chia seeds, and sliced almonds.

These breakfast treats are designed to assist metabolism, boost energy levels, and adhere to the Blood Type O diet guidelines. Savor the path to wellness with filling and delectable breakfasts!

Chapter 4: Lunchtime Favorites

1. Grilled Salmon Salad

Ingredients:

- Mixed salad greens

- 6 oz. salmon fillet

- Halved cherry tomatoes

- Sliced cucumber

- 1/4 cup crumbled feta cheese

- Lemon juice and olive oil for dressing

- To taste, add salt and pepper.

Guidelines:

Sprinkle salt and pepper on the salmon fillet. Grill the salmon until cooked through. Combine the cucumber, cherry tomatoes, and mixed salad greens in a bowl. Top with the grilled salmon. Drizzle with olive oil and lemon juice. Top the salad with feta cheese crumbles.

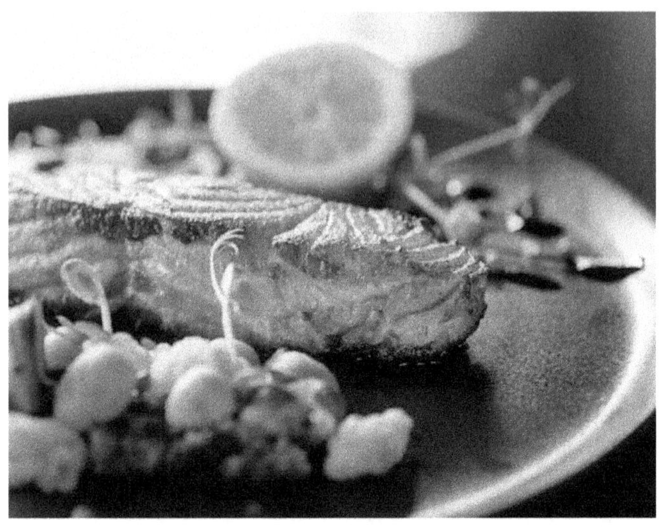

2. Turkey and Avocado Wrap

Ingredients:

- 1 whole grain wrap

- 4 ounces of sliced turkey breast

- 1/2 avocado, sliced

- Mixed greens

- Mustard for dressing

- To taste, add salt and pepper.

Guidelines:

Place the whole grain wrap onto a level surface. Layer mixed greens, avocado slices, and turkey slices. Add pepper and salt for seasoning. To enhance the flavor, drizzle with mustard. Tightly roll the wrap, then slice in half.

3. Lentil Soup with Spinach

Ingredients:

- 1 cup dried green lentils

- 1 chopped onion

- 2 sliced carrots

- 2 chopped celery stalks

- 3 minced garlic cloves

- 1 teaspoon cumin

- 2 cups chopped spinach

- 4 cups vegetable broth

- To taste, add salt and pepper

Guidelines:

Give the lentils a good rinse in cold water. Saute the garlic, celery, carrots, and onions in a pot until tender. Add cumin, lentils, vegetable broth, salt, and pepper. Simmer until lentils are cooked. Add chopped spinach and stir, then cook until it wilts.

Kale and Chicken Caesar Salad

Ingredients:

- 2 cups chopped kale

- 4 ounces sliced grilled chicken breast

- Halved cherry tomatoes

- 1/4 cup Parmesan cheese, grated

- Caesar dressing

- Croutons (optional)

- Sliced lemons for decoration

Guidelines:

Gently massage chopped kale with a bit of olive oil to make it softer. Mix kale, cherry tomatoes, grilled chicken, and Parmesan cheese in a bowl. Drizzle with Caesar dressing. If preferred, add croutons to top. Add lemon wedges as a garnish.

5. Stir-fried Broccoli and Beef

Ingredients:

- 8 ounces lean beef strips

- 2 cups florets of broccoli

- 1 sliced bell pepper

- 2 minced garlic cloves

- 2 tsp. soy sauce

- 1 tablespoon olive oil

- Brown rice for serving

- Sesame seeds for garnish

Guidelines:

Heat the olive oil in a wok over high heat. Stir-fry beef until browned, then set aside. In the same wok, stir-fry broccoli, bell pepper, and garlic until tender-crisp. Return the cooked beef back to the wok. Pour soy sauce into the mixture and toss to coat thoroughly. Top with sesame seeds and serve over brown rice.

6. Greek Yogurt Chicken Salad

Ingredients:

- 1/2 cup Greek yogurt

- 6 ounces grilled, shredded chicken breast

- 2 tablespoons finely chopped red onion

- 1/4 cup diced cucumber

- 1/4 cup cherry tomatoes, halved

- Fresh dill for garnish

- Salt and pepper to taste

Guidelines:

Combine cucumber, cherry tomatoes, red onion, Greek yogurt, and shredded chicken in a bowl. Mix until thoroughly blended. Add pepper and salt for seasoning. Add fresh dill as garnish.

7. Shrimp and Asparagus Stir-fry

Ingredients:

- 1 bunch of asparagus, chopped and trimmed

- 1 bell pepper, sliced

- 8 ounces of peeled and deveined shrimp

- 2 tsp. soy sauce

- 1 tablespoon sesame oil

- 1 tablespoon finely chopped ginger

- Brown rice for serving

Guidelines:

In a wok, heat sesame oil over medium-high heat. Stir-fry shrimp until pink, then put it aside. Stir-fry bell pepper, ginger, and asparagus in the same wok until the veggies are tender-crisp.

Return the cooked shrimp back to the wok. Pour the mixture with soy sauce and toss to coat thoroughly. Serve with brown rice.

8. Kidney Beans with Turkey Chili

Ingredients:

- 1 pound ground turkey

- 1 chopped onion

- 2 minced garlic cloves

- 1 can (15 oz) drained and rinsed kidney beans

- 1 can (14-ounce) diced tomatoes

- 1 cup of tomato sauce

- 2 tablespoons chili powder

- To taste, add salt and pepper

- Greek yogurt for topping

Guidelines:

In a saucepan, cook ground turkey until brown. Add minced garlic and onions, sauté until softened. Stir in kidney beans, chopped tomatoes, tomato sauce, salt, pepper, and chili powder. Simmer for 20 minutes or longer. Top with a generous dollop of Greek yogurt and serve.

9. Turkey Quinoa Bowl with Mushrooms

Ingredients:

- 4 ounces ground turkey

- 1 cup sliced mushrooms

- 1 cup cooked quinoa

- 1/2 cup finely chopped spinach

- 1 tbsp. soy sauce

- 1 tablespoon olive oil

- Sesame seeds for garnish

Guidelines:

Heat olive oil in a skillet over medium heat. Cook the ground turkey until browned. Add mushrooms and sauté until soft. Stir in the soy sauce and chopped spinach. Layer the turkey-mushroom-spinach mixture and cooked quinoa in a bowl. Add sesame seeds as a garnish.

10. Baked Chicken with Sweet Potatoes

Ingredients:

- 1 tablespoon olive oil

- 2 peeled and diced sweet potatoes

- 4 bone-in and skin-on chicken thighs

- 1 tsp. of paprika

- 1 teaspoon garlic powder

- Season with salt and pepper

- Fresh parsley for garnish

Guidelines:

Turn the oven on to 400°F (200°C). Combine the chopped sweet potatoes, olive oil, salt, pepper, paprika, and garlic powder in a bowl. Place the sweet potatoes and chicken thighs on a baking sheet.

Bake the chicken for 35 to 40 minutes, or until it is cooked thoroughly. Before serving, garnish with fresh parsley.

These carefully planned lunches offer filling and delectable options for a midday feast while adhering to the Blood Type O diet's meals. Savor these delicious treats as you progress toward fitness!

Chapter 5: Dinner Creations

1. Grilled Lemon Herb Chicken

Ingredients:

- 4 skinless, boneless chicken breasts
- 1 lemon juice
- 2 tablespoons olive oil
- 2 teaspoons dried thyme
- 2 teaspoon oregano
- To taste, salt and pepper

Guidelines:

Mix lemon juice, olive oil, salt, pepper, oregano, and thyme in a bowl. Marinate the chicken breasts in the mixture for a minimum of 30 minutes. Preheat the grill and cook the chicken for about 6 to 8 minutes on each side, or until it's done.

Quinoa Stuffed Bell Peppers

Ingredients:

- 1 cup cooked quinoa

- 1 pound ground turkey

- 1 chopped onion

- 1 can (15 oz.) of drained and rinsed black beans

- 1 cup tomato sauce

- 4 bell peppers, halved and seeds removed

- 1 teaspoon cumin

- To taste, add salt and pepper

Guidelines:

Turn the oven on to 375°F (190°C). Cook the ground turkey in a skillet until browned. Add chopped onions and sauté until tender. Stir in black beans, tomato sauce, cumin, cooked quinoa, salt, and pepper. Stuff each bell pepper with the quinoa-turkey mixture. Bake the peppers for 25 to 30 minutes, or until they are tender.

3. Salmon and Asparagus Foil Packets

Ingredients:

- 4 salmon fillets

- 1 bunch trimmed asparagus

- Two teaspoons olive oil

- Two minced garlic cloves

- Lemon slices for garnish

- Salt and pepper to taste

Guidelines:

Turn the oven on to 400°F (200°C). Place each salmon fillet on a piece of foil. Position the asparagus around the salmon. Drizzle olive oil on the asparagus and salmon. Add pepper, salt, and minced garlic. Seal the foil packets and bake for 15 to 20 minutes or until the salmon is cooked.

4. Vegetable Stir-Fry with Tofu

Ingredients:

- 2 cups of broccoli florets

- 1 block firm tofu, pressed and cubed

- 1 sliced bell pepper

- 1 julienned carrot

- 1 cup snap peas

- 2 tablespoons soy sauce

- 1 tablespoon of sesame oil

- 1 tablespoon minced ginger

Guidelines:

In a wok, heat the sesame oil over medium-high heat. Stir-fry tofu until golden brown. Add the snap peas, carrot, bell pepper, and broccoli. Stir in the minced ginger and soy sauce. Simmer the vegetables until they are tender-crisp.

5. Baked Turkey and Sweet Potato Casserole

Ingredients:

- 1 pound ground turkey

- 2 peeled and sliced sweet potatoes

- 1 diced onion

- 1 can (14 oz.) of diced tomatoes

- 1 cup chicken broth

- 1 teaspoon paprika

- 1 teaspoon powdered garlic

- To taste, add salt and pepper.

Guidelines:

Turn the oven on to 375°F (190°C). Cook the ground turkey in a skillet until browned. Add chopped onions and sauté until tender. Layer slices of sweet potato in a baking tray. Top with diced tomatoes and cooked turkey. Combine the chicken broth, salt, pepper, paprika, and garlic powder; drizzle it over the casserole. Bake for 35 to 40 minutes, or until sweet potatoes are soft.

6. Shrimp and Quinoa Bowl

Ingredients:

- 1 cup cooked quinoa

- 1/2 cup halved cherry tomatoes

- 1 cup broccoli florets

- 8 oz. peeled and deveined shrimp

- 1 tablespoon olive oil

- A sprinkling of sesame seeds

Guidelines:

In a skillet, heat the olive oil over medium-high heat. Add shrimp and stir-fry until pink. Add the broccoli and cook until tender-crisp. Stir in cherry tomatoes and cooked quinoa. Drizzle soy sauce over the mixture and toss to coat thoroughly. Add sesame seeds as a garnish.

7. Mushroom and Spinach Stuffed Chicken

Ingredients:

- 4 skinless, boneless chicken breasts

- 1 cup chopped mushrooms

- 1 cup of chopped spinach

- 1/4 cup crumbled feta cheese

- 2 tsp. olive oil

- 2 minced garlic cloves

- To taste, add salt and pepper.

Guidelines:

Turn the oven on to 375°F (190°C). Sauté garlic and mushrooms in olive oil in a skillet until the mushrooms are tender. Add chopped spinach and stir until it wilts. Slice a pocket in each chicken breast, then fill it with the mushroom-spinach mixture. Place stuffed chicken breasts in a baking dish. Bake for 25 to 30 minutes, or until the chicken is thoroughly cooked.

8. Turkey and Vegetable Skewers

Ingredients:

- 1 pound turkey breast, cubed

- Assorted colored bell peppers, chopped into chunks

- Sliced zucchini

- Cherry tomatoes

- 2 tablespoons olive oil

- 1 teaspoon powdered garlic

- 1 teaspoon dried oregano

- To taste, add salt and pepper.

Guidelines:

Preheat the grill or grill pan. Thread cherry tomatoes, bell peppers, zucchini, and turkey onto skewers. Combine olive oil, salt, pepper, oregano, and garlic powder in a bowl. Brush the skewers with the oil mixture. Grill for 10 to 15 minutes, flipping it occasionally, until the turkey is thoroughly cooked.

9. Eggplant and Tomato Stew

Ingredients:

- 1 large diced eggplant

- 1 diced onion

- 2 cloves garlic, minced

- 1 can (14-oz) chopped tomatoes

- 1 cup of vegetable broth

- 1 teaspoon dried oregano

- 1 teaspoon dried basil

- To taste, add salt and pepper.

Guidelines:

Sauté onions and garlic in a pot until softened. Add the chopped eggplant and cook until it begins to get tender. Stir in diced tomatoes, salt, pepper, oregano, basil, and vegetable broth. Simmer for 20 to 25 minutes or until the eggplant is tender.

10. Tuna and Avocado Salad

Ingredients:

- 2 cans (5 oz. each) drained tuna
- 2 diced avocados
- 1 diced cucumber
- 1/4 cup finely sliced red onion
- 2 teaspoons olive oil
- 1 lemon's juice
- To taste, add salt and pepper.

Guidelines:

Mix diced avocados, diced cucumber, diced red onion, and drained tuna in a bowl. Drizzle with lemon juice and olive oil.

Toss gently until thoroughly mixed. Add pepper and salt for seasoning.

These dinner recipes offer a range of tasty and nourishing options to promote your well-being, while adhering to the principles of the Blood Type O diet.

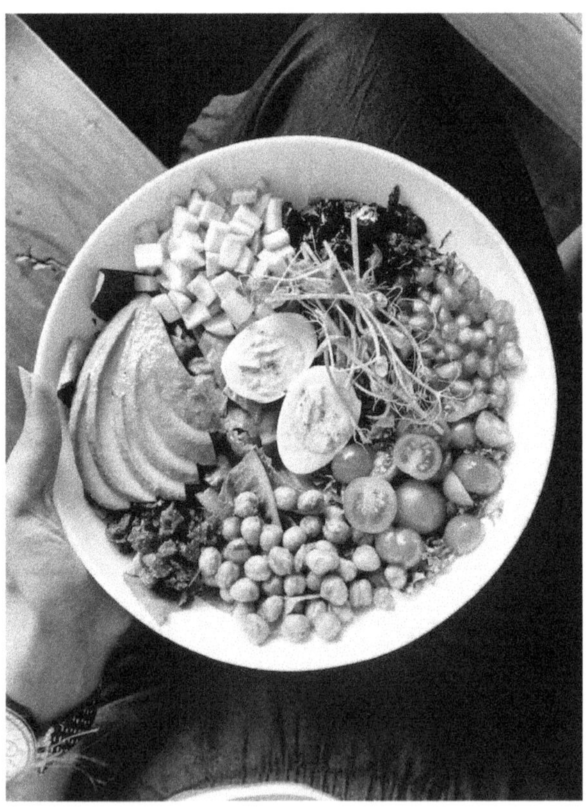

Chapter 6: Sides and Snacks

1. Turkey Bacon with Roasted Brussels sprouts

Ingredients:

- 1 pound halved Brussels sprouts -

- 4 chopped slices of turkey bacon

- 2 tsp. olive oil

- 1 teaspoon powdered garlic

- To taste, add salt and pepper.

Guidelines:

Turn the oven on to 400°F (200°C). Toss olive oil, salt, pepper, and garlic powder with the turkey bacon and Brussels sprouts. Place the mixture onto a baking sheet. Roast Brussels sprouts for 20 to 25 minutes, or until they turn golden brown.

2. Cucumber and Tomato Salad

Ingredients:

- 2 sliced cucumbers

- 1 cup halved cherry tomatoes

- 1/4 cup finely chopped red onion

- 2 teaspoons olive oil

- 1 tsp. balsamic vinegar

- Fresh basil for garnish

- To taste, add salt and pepper

Guidelines:

Mix chopped red onion, cherry tomatoes, and cucumber slices in a bowl. Drizzle with balsamic vinegar and olive oil. Toss to coat thoroughly. Add fresh basil as a garnish. Add pepper and salt for seasoning.

3. Stuffed Grape Leaves with Ground Turkey

Ingredients:

- 1 jar of drained grape leaves

- 1 cup cooked quinoa

- 1/4 cup pine nuts

- 2 tablespoons lemon juice

- 1/2 pound ground turkey

- 1 teaspoon of dried dill

- Salt and pepper to taste

Guidelines:

Cook the ground turkey in a skillet until browned. Combine cooked ground turkey, quinoa, pine nuts, dried dill, lemon juice, salt, and pepper in a bowl. Scoop out a portion of the mixture onto each grape leaf, then tightly roll it up. Serve chilled.

4. Baked Sweet Potato Fries

Ingredients:

- 1 teaspoon paprika

- 2 tablespoons olive oil

- 2 sweet potatoes, cut into fries

- 1 teaspoon powdered garlic

- To taste, add salt and pepper.

Guidelines:

Turn the oven on to 425°F (220°C). Toss olive oil, salt, pepper, paprika, and garlic powder with sweet potato fries. Layer the fries on a baking sheet. Bake the fries for 20 to 25 minutes, or until they are crispy.

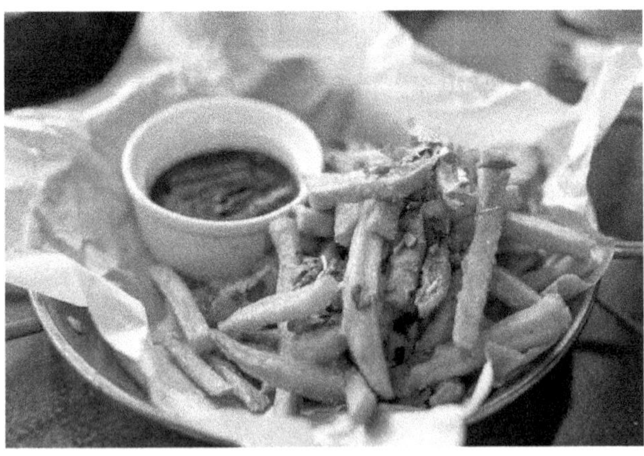

5. Guacamole with Jicama Sticks

Ingredients:

- 3 avocados, mashed

- 1 diced tomato

- 1/4 cup finely chopped red onion

- 1/4 cup chopped cilantro

- 1 lime's juice

- Jicama sticks for dipping

- Salt and pepper to taste

Guidelines:

Combine diced tomato, chopped red onion, cilantro, lime juice, and mashed avocados in a bowl. Mix until thoroughly combined. Add pepper and salt for seasoning. Serve with jicama sticks for dipping.

Greek Hummus with Veggie Sticks

Ingredients:

- 1 can (15 oz.) drained chickpeas

- 2 tablespoons olive oil

- 2 tablespoons tahini

- 1 lemon's juice

- 1 minced clove garlic

- 1/2 teaspoon oregano, dried

- Carrot and cucumber sticks for dipping

Guidelines:

Blend the chickpeas, tahini, olive oil, lemon juice, minced garlic, and dried oregano in a food processor until smooth. To taste, add salt and pepper for seasoning. Serve with cucumber and carrot sticks for dipping.

7. Kale Chips with Sea Salt

Ingredients:

- 1 bunch kale, stems removed and torn into pieces

- 2 tablespoons olive oil

- Sea salt to taste

Guidelines:

Preheat the oven to 350°F (175°C). Toss kale pieces with olive oil. Layer the kale on a baking sheet. Add a dash of sea salt. Bake the kale for10 to 15 minutes, or until crispy.

8. Mango Salsa with Plantain Chips

Ingredients:

- 2 mangoes, diced

- 1/4 cup red onion, finely chopped

- 1 jalapeño, seeded and finely chopped

- 1/4 cup finely chopped fresh cilantro

- 1 lime's juice

- Plantain chips for dipping

- Salt and pepper to taste

Guidelines:

Combine chopped red onion, jalapeño, cilantro, lime juice, and diced mangoes in a bowl. Mix until thoroughly combined.

Add pepper and salt to seasoning. Accompany with plantain chips for dipping.

9. Turkey Lettuce Wraps

Ingredients:

- 1 pound of ground turkey

- 1 tablespoon olive oil

- 1 chopped onion

- 1 bell pepper, chopped

- 1/4 cup water chestnuts, chopped

- Butter lettuce leaves for wrapping

- Hoisin sauce for drizzling

Guidelines:

In a skillet, heat olive oil over medium heat. Cook ground turkey until browned. Add water chestnuts, bell peppers, and sliced onions. Stir until vegetables are softened. Spoon the turkey mixture onto butter lettuce leaves. Drizzle with hoisin sauce.

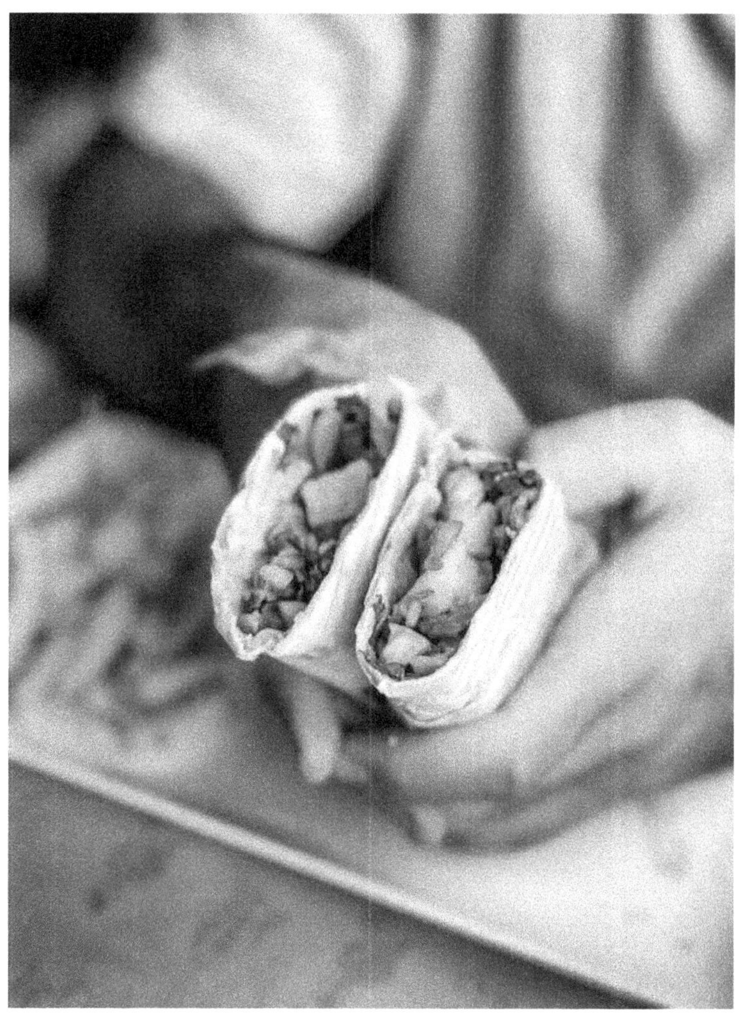

10. Sesame Seed Snap Peas

Ingredients:

- 2 cups of trimmed snap peas

- 1 tablespoon sesame oil

- 1 tablespoon sesame seeds

- To taste, add salt and pepper.

Guidelines

In a pan, heat sesame oil over a medium-high heat. Add snap peas and cook until tender-crisp. Top the snap peas with sesame seeds. Add pepper and salt for seasoning.

These sides and snacks are crafted with the principles of the Blood Type O diet in mind, providing a variety of flavors and textures to enhance your eating experience while supporting your well-being. Enjoy these delicious and nutritious options!

Chapter 7: Refreshing Smoothies

1. Tropical Green Smoothie

Ingredients:

- 1/2 cup pineapple chunks

- 1 cup kale leaves, stems removed

- 1/2 banana

- 1/2 avocado

- 1 cup coconut water

- Ice cubes, if desired

Guidelines:

Put kale, avocado, banana, pineapple, and coconut water in a blender. Blend until smooth. Add ice cubes if desired and blend once more. Pour into a glass and savor the delicious tropical green flavor.

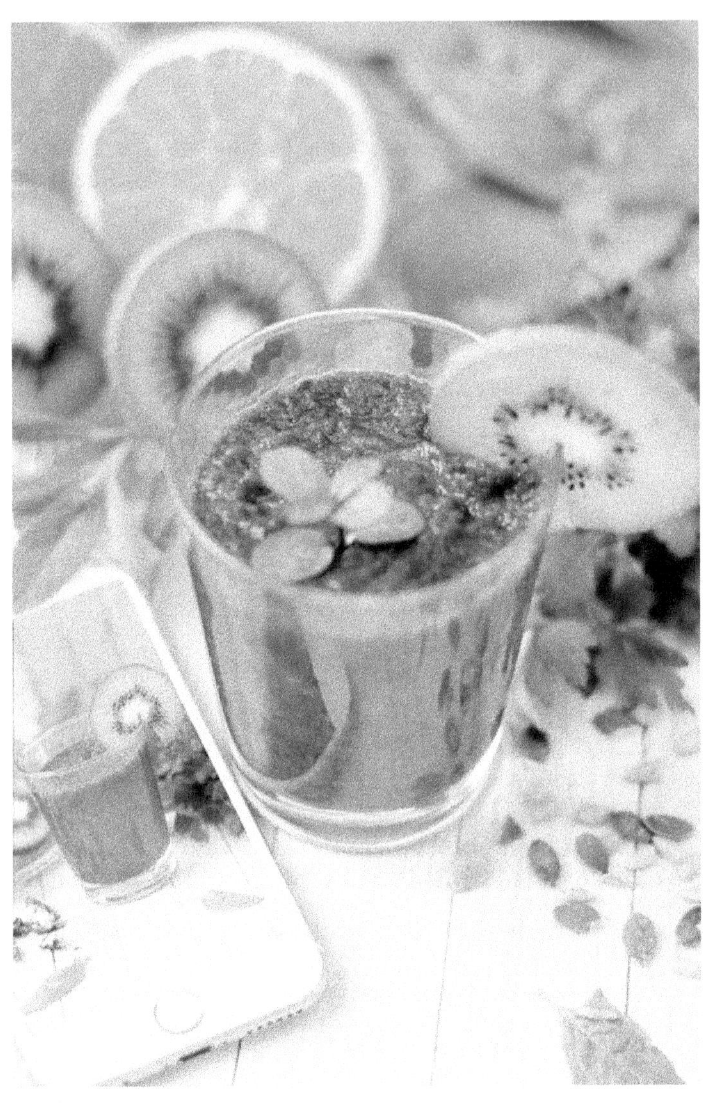

2. Berry Protein Blast

Ingredients:

- 1/2 cup mixed berries (strawberries, raspberries, and blueberries)

- 1/2 banana

- 1/2 cup Greek yogurt

- 1 scoop (plant-based) protein powder

- 1 cup almond milk

- Chia seeds, as a garnish (optional)

Guidelines

Put mixed berries, banana, Greek yogurt, almond milk, and protein powder in a blender. Blend until smooth. Pour into a glass, and if desired, top with chia seeds. Enjoy this protein-rich berry treat.

3. Citrus Mint Refresher

Ingredients:

- 1 orange, segmented and peeled

- 1/2 grapefruit, segmented and peeled

- 1/2 lime juiced

- Scoop of mint leaves that are fresh

- 1 tablespoon honey, if desired

- Ice cubes, if desired

Guidelines.

Put orange, grapefruit, lime juice, and fresh mint leaves in a blender. Blend until smooth. If preferred, add honey for sweetness. If you want a cold beverage, add ice cubes. Transfer to a glass and savor the deliciously zesty citrus flavor.

4. Creamy Almond Butter Banana Smoothie

Ingredients:

- 2 bananas

- 2 tsp. almond butter

- 1/2 cup almond milk

- 1/2 teaspoon vanilla extract

- A tiny pinch of cinnamon

- Ice cubes, if desired

Guidelines:

Put bananas, almond milk, almond butter, cinnamon, and vanilla extract in a blender. Then blend until smooth. To achieve a colder consistency, add ice cubes. Pour into a glass and enjoy the deliciously creamy almond flavor.

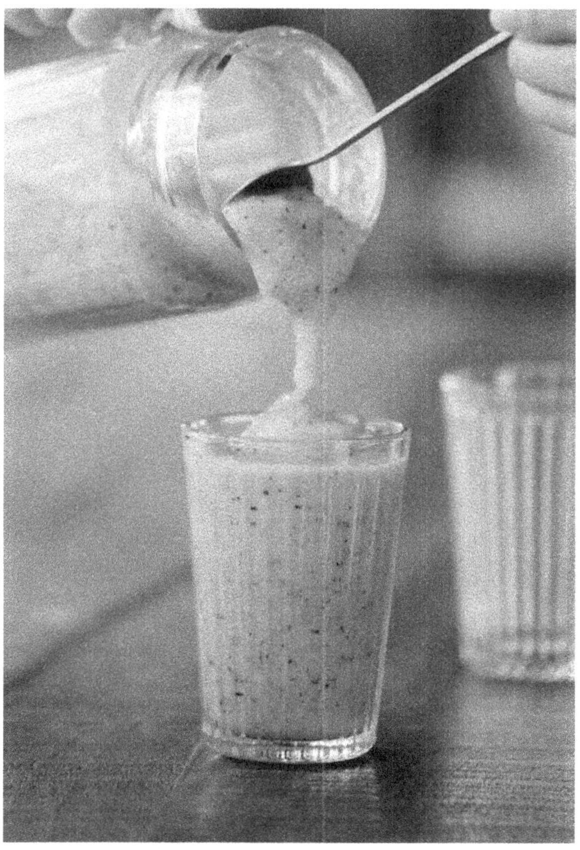

5. Pomegranate Blueberry Bliss

Ingredients:

- 1/2 cup pomegranate seeds

- 1/2 cup blueberries

- 1/2 cup plain yogurt (sheep or goat milk preferably)

- 1 tablespoon flax seeds

- 1/2 cup water

- Ice cubes, if desired

Guidelines:

Put the blueberries, yogurt, water, flaxseeds, and pomegranate seeds in a blender. Then blend until smooth. If you prefer your smoothie cold, add some ice cubes. Pour into a glass and savor the delight of rich antioxidant content.

6. Mango Ginger Energizer

Ingredients:

- 1/2 teaspoon grated ginger

- 1/2 cup coconut water

- 1/2 cup water

- 1 cup mango chunks

- Fresh lime juice, to taste

- Ice cubes, if desired

Guidelines:

Put the mango chunks, grated ginger, water, coconut water, and lime juice in a blender. Then blend until smooth. Add ice cubes for a chilly, refreshing touch. Pour into a glass and savor this revitalizing mixture.

7. Spinach and Pineapple Detox Smoothie

Ingredients:

- 1 cup pineapple chunk

- Two cups spinach leaves, fresh

- 1/2 cucumbers, peeled and sliced

- 1/2 lemon, juiced

- 1 tsp. chia seeds

- Ice cubes, if desired

Guidelines:

Put spinach, pineapple, cucumber, lemon juice, and chia seeds in a blender. Blend until smooth. Add ice cubes for a cool, cleansing feeling. Pour into a glass and savor the delicious green flavor.

8. Anti-Inflammatory Turmeric Mango Smoothie

Ingredients:

- 1/2 teaspoon powdered turmeric
- 1 cup mango chunks
- 1/2 teaspoon grated fresh turmeric
- 1/2 cup coconut milk
- 1/2 cup of water
- Honey to taste (optional)
- Ice cubes, if desired

Guidelines:

Put mango chunks, fresh turmeric, powdered turmeric, coconut milk, water, and honey in a blender. Blend until smooth. Include ice cubes for a cool variation. Pour into a glass and savor this anti-inflammatory elixir

9. Cherry Almond Protein Smoothie

Ingredients:

- 1/2 cup pitted cherries

- 1/2 half banana

- 1/4 cup almonds

- 1 scoop protein powder (rice or pea protein)

- 1 cup almond milk

- Ice cubes, if desired

Guidelines:

Put the almonds, banana, cherries, protein powder, and almond milk in a blender. Blend until smooth. For a refreshing and satisfying texture, add ice cubes. Pour into a glass and savor the cherry-almond protein boost.

10. Coconut Berry Hydration Smoothie

Ingredients:

- 1/2 cup mixed berries (raspberries, blueberries, strawberries)
- 1/2 cup coconut water
- 1/2 cup water
- 1/2 lime, juiced
- 1 tablespoon chia seeds
- Ice cubes, if desired

Guidelines:

Combine mixed berries, water, coconut water, lime juice, and chia seeds in a blender. Blend until smooth. Add ice cubes for a revitalizing hydration boost. Pour into a glass and savor the mix of tropical berries.

These cool smoothies boost your wellbeing while providing a wonderful variety of flavors and are created with the Blood Type O diet in mind. Savor these tasty and nutrient-dense smoothies as a part of your healthy diet!

Chapter 8: Desserts for Blood Type O

1. Berry Chia Pudding Parfait

Ingredients:

- 1/4 cup chia seeds

- 1/2 cup of mixed berries (strawberries, blueberries raspberries)

- 1 cup almond milk

- 1 teaspoon vanilla extract

- 1 tablespoon chopped nuts (either almonds or walnuts

Guidelines:

Combine almond milk, vanilla extract, and chia seeds in a bowl. Refrigerate until the chia seeds absorb the liquid, which should take at least two hours or overnight.

Layer chia pudding with mixed berries in a glass. Repeat the layers, then sprinkle chopped nuts on top. Savor this tasty and nourishing parfait.

2. Avocado Chocolate Mousse

Ingredients:

- 1/4 cup cocoa powder

- 2 ripe avocados

- 1 teaspoon vanilla extract

- 1/4 cup maple syrup

- A pinch of sea salt

- Berries as a garnish

Guidelines:

Put avocados, sea salt, vanilla extract, maple syrup, and cocoa powder in a blender. Blend until creamy and smooth. Refrigerate for a minimum of 30 minutes. Spoon the chocolate mousse into bowls and top with fresh berries as garnish.

3. Coconut Almond Energy Bites

Ingredients:

- 1 cup coconut shreds

- 1/2 cup almond butter

- 1/4 cup almonds, chopped

- 1/4 cup honey

- 1/2 teaspoon vanilla extract

- A dash of sea salt

Guidelines:

Mix chopped almonds, honey, almond butter, shredded coconut, vanilla extract, and sea salt in a bowl. Refrigerate for 30 minutes. Shape the mixture into small bites. Store in the refrigerator and enjoy these energy-packed treats.

4. Cinnamon Baked Apples

Ingredients:

- 1 tablespoon melted coconut oil

- 1 teaspoon cinnamon

- 2 cored and sliced apples

- 1 tablespoon of honey

- Chopped walnuts for garnish

Guidelines:

Turn the oven on to 375°F (190°C). In a bowl, toss apple slices with honey, cinnamon, and melted coconut oil. Layer the apple slices on a baking sheet. Bake for 20 to 25 minutes, or until the apples are soft. Sprinkle chopped walnuts on top, then serve hot.

5. Banana Almond Ice Cream

Ingredients:

- 2 ripe banana, frozen and sliced

- 2 tsp. almond butter

- 1/2 a teaspoon vanilla extract

- Garnish with almond slices

Guidelines:

Put almond butter, vanilla extract, and frozen banana slices in a blender. Blend until creamy and smooth. Scoop into dishes and garnish with almond slices. Savor this guilt-free banana almond ice cream.

6. Pumpkin Spice Chia Pudding

Ingredients:

- 1/4 cup chia seeds

- 1 cup coconut milk

- 1/4 cup pumpkin puree

- 1 tsp. maple syrup

- 1/2 teaspoon of spiced pumpkin

- Pecans as garnish

Guidelines:

Mix chia seeds, maple syrup, pumpkin puree, coconut milk, and pumpkin spice in a bowl. Refrigerate for a minimum of 2 hours, or until the liquid is absorbed by the chia seeds. Scoop the pudding into bowls and sprinkle pecans on top. Enjoy the delicious flavor of pumpkin spice.

7. Greek Yogurt and Honey Parfait

Ingredients:

- 1 cup Greek yogurt

- 1/4 cup granola

- 2 teaspoons honey

- Mixed berries for topping

Guidelines:

Layer honey and Greek yogurt into a glass. Top with mixed berries and granola. Repeat the layers again. Top with a bit more honey and serve this easy yet filling parfait.

8. Almond Flour Banana Bread

Ingredients:

- 2 ripe banana, mashed

- 2 eggs

- 1/4 cup melted coconut oil

- 1/2 teaspoon baking soda

- 1 teaspoon vanilla extract

- 2 cups almond flour

- A pinch of salt

- Chopped dark chocolate (optional) for extra richness

Guidelines:

Preheat the oven to 350°F (175°C). Mix eggs, melted coconut oil, vanilla extract, and mashed bananas in a bowl. Add salt, baking soda, and almond flour. Mix well until thoroughly blended. If preferred, fold in chopped dark chocolate.

Pour batter into an oiled loaf pan. Bake for 40 to 45 minutes, or until a toothpick comes out clean. Let it cool before cutting into slices and enjoying this almond flour banana bread.

9. Cocoa-Dusted Almonds

Ingredients:

- 1 cup raw almonds
- 1 tablespoon powdered cocoa
- 1 spoonful of maple syrup
- A dash of sea salt

Guidelines:

Preheat the oven to 350°F (175°C). Toss sea salt, maple syrup, and cocoa powder with raw almonds in a bowl. Layer the almonds on a baking tray. Bake, stirring periodically, for 12 to 15 minutes.

Allow to cool before savoring these almonds sprinkled with cocoa.

10. Vanilla Berry Sorbet

Ingredients:

- 1 tablespoon honey

- 1 teaspoon vanilla extract

- 2 cups mixed berries (strawberries, blueberries, raspberries)

- Fresh mint leaves for garnish

Guidelines:

Put mixed berries, honey, and vanilla extract in a blender. Blend until smooth. Pour the mixture into a shallow dish and freeze for a minimum of 4 hours, stirring every hour. Scoop into bowls, top with mint leaves, and enjoy this sorbet that sweetens naturally.

These dessert recipes offer a variety of delectable options to fulfill your sweet craving while adhering to your dietary preferences, and they are created with the Blood Type O diet's principle in mind. Savor these sweet treats as part of a well-rounded, health-conscious dessert menu!

Meal Plan and Tips for Blood Type O Diet

14-Days Meal Plan

DAY 1

Breakfast: Scrambled eggs with spinach and turkey sausage

Lunch: Grilled chicken salad with mixed greens, tomatoes, and olive oil dressing

Dinner: Baked salmon with steamed broccoli and quinoa

DAY 2

Breakfast: Greek yogurt with berries and a drizzle of chia seeds

Lunch: Turkey lettuce wraps with avocado and salsa

Dinner: Stir-fried shrimp with veggies (bell peppers, broccoli, onions) over brown rice

DAY 3

Breakfast: Omelet with mushrooms, onions, and feta cheese

Lunch: Quinoa salad with diced chicken, cherry tomatoes, and cucumber

Dinner: Baked cod with sweet potato wedges and asparagus

DAY 4

Breakfast: Smoothie with banana, almond milk, spinach, and protein powder

Lunch: Lentil soup with a side of mixed greens

Dinner: Turkey and vegetable kebabs with a side of cauliflower rice

---

DAY 5

Breakfast: Almond flour pancakes with fresh berries and a drizzle of honey

Lunch: Tuna salad with mixed greens, olives, and a lemon vinaigrette

Dinner: Grilled lamb chops with roasted Brussels sprouts and quinoa

---

DAY 6

Breakfast: Cottage cheese with sliced pineapple and a handful of walnuts

Lunch: Stir-fried chicken and vegetables with ginger and soy sauce over rice noodles

Dinner: Baked chicken thighs with sweet potato mash and green beans

DAY 7

Breakfast: Smoked salmon with whole grain toast and avocado

Lunch: Spinach and feta stuffed chicken breast with a side of roasted veggies

Dinner: Shrimp and vegetable curry with cauliflower rice

DAY 8

Breakfast: Almond milk-based chia seed pudding topped with sliced strawberries

Lunch: Avocado and turkey wrap with a side of raw carrot sticks

Dinner: Baked tilapia with quinoa and mixed green salad

DAY 9

Breakfast: Banana and almond butter smoothie

Lunch: Lentils and vegetables stew accompanied with a side of mixed berries

Dinner: Stir-fried broccoli and beef over brown rice

DAY 10

Breakfast: Scrambled eggs with sautéed spinach and cherry tomatoes

Lunch: Greek salad with grilled chicken and a lemon-oregano dressing

Dinner: Roasted sweet potatoes and green beans accompanied with baked halibut

DAY 11

Breakfast: Oatmeal with sliced apples, cinnamon, and a dollop of Greek yogurt

Lunch: Turkey and Vegetable kebabs with a side of quinoa

Dinner: Stir-fried shrimp with broccoli, bell peppers, and snap peas over cauliflower rice

DAY 12

Breakfast: Smoothie bowl with mixed berries, banana, and granola

Lunch: Chickpea and vegetable curry with a side of steamed kale

Dinner: Grilled chicken with a side of asparagus and sweet potato wedges

DAY 13

Breakfast: Whole grain toast with avocado and poached eggs

Lunch: Tuna and white bean salad with mixed greens

Dinner: Baked cod with quinoa and side of roasted Brussels sprouts

DAY 14

Breakfast: Cottage cheese with sliced peaches and a handful of almonds

Lunch: Stir-fried chicken and vegetables with cashews over brown rice

Dinner: Turkey chili with kidney beans and a side of mixed green salad

Feel free to mix and match meals to suit your tastes, but for individualized advice, think about speaking with a nutritionist or healthcare provider. Adapt serving sizes to your specific energy needs and objectives. Do not forget to drink plenty of water or herbal teas to stay hydrated during the day. Have fun with your Blood Type O meal plan!

Grocery Shopping Guide

This guide will assist you to choose foods that fits with the principles of the Blood Type O diet, focusing on lean proteins, vegetables, fruits, and other beneficial options.

PROTEINS

1. Lean Meats:

- Grass-fed beef
- Lamb
- Turkey
- Venison

2. Seafood:

- Salmon
- Cod
- Halibut
- Sardines
- Shrimp

3. Poultry:

- Chicken

- Turkey

4. Dairy:

- Greek yogurt (preferably goat or sheep milk)

- Feta cheese

- Mozzarella cheese (in moderation)

- Cottage cheese (in moderation)

VEGETABLES

1. Leafy Greens:

- Kale

- Spinach

- Romaine lettuce

- Swiss chard

2. Cruciferous Vegetables:

- Broccoli

- Brussels sprouts

- Cauliflower

3. Root Vegetables:

- Sweet potatoes

- Carrots

- Beets

4. Other Vegetables:

- Bell peppers

- Onions

- Garlic

- Cucumbers

FRUITS

1. Berries:

- Blueberries
- Strawberries
- Blackberries

2. Other Fruits:

- Pineapple
- Cherries
- Plums

GRAINS AND LEGUMES

1. Quinoa
2. Brown rice
3. Lentils

4. Avoid:

- Wheat products
- Corn

NUTS AND SEEDS

1. Almonds
2. Walnuts
3. Chia seeds
4. Flaxseeds

HEALTHY FATS

1. Olive oil
2. Avocado oil
3. Flaxseed oil

HERBS AND SPICES

1. Turmeric
2. Ginger
3. Rosemary
4. Thyme
5. Garlic powder

BEVERAGES

1. Green tea

2. Herbal teas

3. Water with lemon

SWEETENERS

1. Honey (in moderation)

2. Maple syrup (in moderation)

MISCELLANEOUS

1. Eggs (free-range, organic)

2. Coconut milk (unsweetened)

3. Coconut water

4. Dark chocolate (in moderation, at least 70% cocoa)

Tips for Shopping

1. Choose organic options whenever possible.

2. Select fresh, local produce for optimal nutrients.

3. Read labels to avoid additives, preservatives, and artificial ingredients.

4. Buy in-season fruits and vegetables for better taste and affordability.

5. Opt for grass-fed and free-range meats for higher nutrient content.

Foods to Limit or Avoid

1. Dairy (except those mentioned above)

2. Wheat and gluten-containing products

3. Corn and corn products

4. Kidney beans and lentils (in moderation)

5. Avoid processed and highly sugary foods.

Conclusion

The Blood Type O Cookbook is a bright spot in the colorful tapestry of culinary adventure, showing the way to health, energy, and deliciousness. As we get to the end of this culinary adventure journey specifically for Blood Type O individuals, we honor the harmonious union of taste and nutrition.

Every recipe has a symphony of flavors that are specifically tailored to meet the requirements of Blood Type O, from the crisp crunch of fresh vegetables to the sizzling pan-seared proteins. Every component has been thoughtfully selected for its overall health benefits in addition to its flavor.

This cookbook is an ode to the transforming power of mindful eating, not merely a compilation of recipes. It's a celebration of the relationship that exists between the energy we use and the ingredients we choose. The tales exchanged, the aromas emanating from the kitchen, and the tastes tantalizing your taste buds are all pieces of a narrative that goes beyond simple nourishment.

May the Blood Type O Cookbook be your dependable guide and companion as you set out on your gastronomic adventure, helping you to live a distinctive lifestyle. Savor the satisfaction of preparing meals that uplift your soul as much as your body. Learn how to make every meal a celebration of strength, health, and life itself via the pages of this cookbook.

So, my dear reader, may this cookbook be the start of a flavorful and exciting chapter in your culinary adventure. Savor every mouthful and treasure every chapter. Cheers to a life full of healthy decisions, dancing flavors, and an energized, invigorated you.

Happy Cooking!

Weekly meal planner journal

Weekly Meal Planner
Journal

Dates:

	BREAKFAST	LUNCH	DINNER	SNACKS
MON				
TUE				
WED				
THU				
FRI				
SAT				
SUN				

Shopping list

NOTES

Weekly Meal Planner Journal

Dates:

	BREAKFAST	LUNCH	DINNER	SNACKS
MON				
TUE				
WED				
THU				
FRI				
SAT				
SUN				

Shopping list

NOTES

Weekly Meal Planner Journal

Dates:

	BREAKFAST	LUNCH	DINNER	SNACKS
MON				
TUE				
WED				
THU				
FRI				
SAT				
SUN				

Shopping list

NOTES

Weekly Meal Planner Journal

Dates:

	BREAKFAST	LUNCH	DINNER	SNACKS
MON				
TUE				
WED				
THU				
FRI				
SAT				
SUN				

Shopping list

NOTES